First Published in 2011
JD Wildi Publishing
South Wales UK

Text copyright © DebbieWildi
E-mail: debbie@truerelax.co.uk
www.truerelax.co.uk

ISBN 978-0-9568513-0-7

Printed in the UK by
Lightning Source UK Ltd.
Registered in England and Wales
Company number 4042196
Registered office 5 New Street Square, London, EC4A 3TW

For Ollie, Roux and all the children who ever touched my life.

Testimonials taken from children, parents and teachers who use Mini Relax

"Since Lily has been using the book and CD, she hasn't had one bad dream or bad night's sleep. It's worked like magic!"
Cassie (parent of 4 year old)

"This book is lovely, my two often now ask for it before bed. I honestly don't hear a peep from them after they go to sleep, and they sleep really deeply."
Stephanie (parent of 5 and 6 year olds)

"I felt so calm, as if I was flying when Debbie talked us through the story."
Rhian aged 7yrs

"I feel happy and like the noises in my head have stopped. Its magic I think."
Craig aged 6 yrs (suffers with Aspergers Syndrome)

"I feel really proud of myself. I felt so relaxed and quiet. I didn't think that would happen."
Bronwyn aged 10yrs

"When Debbie told us the story of floating on the cloud, I had my eyes closed and felt like I was flying. I was all happy and warm"
Daniel aged 4yrs

"A completely different approach to gaining children's attention. The children were engrossed, calm and content. A valuable all round experience!"
Ms S Williams - Llanilltud Fawr Primary and Nursery School

'Debbie's wonderful techniques can be used by children, at any time of day and in any venue. The simple instructions make relaxation tools very easy to learn in a fun way. As a mother, I would recommend this book to teach our children coping strategies at times when they are nervous or feel vulnerable. On a professional level, children have many pressures put on them by society, if schools taught the techniques used within this book then many children and young people would be more confident to know how to reduce periods of stress in their lives.'
Nadia Stanton BA (hons), I.H.B.C., Cert ed. Coaching & Mentoring
Youth development officer- Vale of Glamorgan council

About the Author

Debbie Wildi lives with her husband and two boys in the Vale of Glamorgan, UK. She has worked with children for most of her life in various ways; teaching them, entertaining them, as well as raising them, and has used her Kiddie calmer techniques and Dreamtime stories to calm children in her care for 22 years.

Debbie has encouraged her own children to use them too, as she knows first hand the debilitating experience of a restless child at night. Neither of her children were sleepers until they became old enough to understand the relaxation techniques and dreamtime stories she created. Once she realised she could use these techniques on her own young toddlers she went from blearily surviving on 3 hours sleep a night to a completely life changing 8 hours. She now teaches *Mini Relax* and *Teen Relax* classes for children of all ages in schools, centres and workshops.

The techniques and stories have been used so successfully here in the UK, that Debbie won the Welsh Spiritual Connection award for her relaxation classes, as well as Best Author award for this book.

For more information on Mini Relax, or to purchase the CD, or teachers programme go to www.truerelax.co.uk

Contents

Introduction

The limitless imagination of a child is such a gift isn't it?
Have you ever seen the wonder in a child's eyes as a sock magically transforms into a puppet, or the excitement build as you tell them their bedtime story?
Turning fantasy into reality during relaxation means the possibilities of stretching their imagination are endless.

This book contains simple and fun ways to help children relax by using their imagination. The kiddie calmers are easy techniques which will instantly calm them, diffuse anger in seconds and unwind their mind, whilst the popular dreamtime stories are tales that they love to listen to and become involved in.

This is a chance to use their minds to take them to an enchanting, tranquil place. It is a great relaxation tool, and a moment to rest their delicate minds from the busy stresses and strains of everyday life.
I have used these techniques for years with my own children, as well as others, and they really do transform bedtime into an enjoyable time to unwind - whilst encouraging sharing and bonding between the reader and child.

Their little brains are active all day every day, and many of them do not know how to switch off at bedtime. The kiddie calmers and dreamtime stories are designed to induce a feeling of calm. Whether they are to be used in the evening, or simply when your child needs some quiet time, I can guarantee that they will be enjoyed over and over for years to come.

Children love to go off into another world in their beautiful heads; climb a beanstalk, spread their imaginary wings and fly. Let's help them get there!

How to use this book

The idea is that this book is read to your child/ren during quiet time, then as they become familiar with the calmers and stories they will be able to remember them at will and take themselves off on a journey in their mind on their own if they wish.

The Kiddie calmers at the start of the book can be used prior to a dreamtime story, or, used separately whenever your child needs some extra calm and focus. They will help them relax and generally bring a wonderful sense of well-being. These are 'easy to learn' breathing techniques that will centre your little one and bring instant relaxation.

I have purposefully designed these to be fun, and your child will love to practice them again and again. They can be carried out anywhere in a short space of time and have worked on adults for many years; why not teach them to our beautiful children? They need the benefits just as much as we do, if not more.

The Dreamtime stories are tales that are read slowly and gently.
As you talk your child through the story they imagine they are taking part in it. It is a wonderful process of bonding between you and your children, and a fantastic confidence builder as they realise they can do this alone once they come to know their favourite stories.

It is important to remember that sometimes they will not want to close their eyes and will wish to watch you as you read. This is fine, do not push your little one/s, let them guide you.

Sometimes they will wish to act out the character and will not want to sit still at all. Go with the flow, the stories can be just as relaxing to gently act out (for example they can lay on the floor/bed and slowly move their butterfly wings, or climb the ladder in the sky to lay on the fluffy cloud). Let them try out different ways of using the stories… eventually most children naturally choose to just lie or sit and close their eyes and listen. However I know some children in the classroom setting who have always preferred to just watch me read the stories and they never fail to become just as relaxed and calm as their peers. The lesson here is to gently guide the child, not force them to relax.

I keep the stories short as attention may wander and we do not want this relaxation time to feel like a chore. It should be something that they look forward to, an enjoyable quest for quiet time, or a bedtime story with a difference!

>>

Make them comfortable, turn off televisions, game consoles etc. Then use their favourite calmer if you feel the need. Do it together maybe? Or go straight to their preferred story. Ask your child to close their eyes if they wish to and read it to them in a soft voice.

Your child will absolutely love their new way of spending story time, and the best part is knowing they are doing it themselves. They are cleverly using the power of their mind to be transported into their very own wonderland just by using their imagination. When they realise the power they have in their own mind the confidence they have in themselves soars... It really does.

Children will gently fall into that sweet feeling of relaxation and lay ready for sleep feeling warm and cosy, relaxed and peace.

Night terrors become a thing of the past, and parents/carers always state that their child looks forward to bedtime when they know a dreamtime story is coming. Studies have shown that a child sleeps much more deeply following a dreamtime story.

The Science behind it

When we listen to a guided visualisation the human brain descends quickly into what is called the Theta brainwave state - a state of pure relaxation. When we are in Theta we feel completely relaxed and our brain is getting ready to descend into the Delta state (the state of sleep).

If we are in the Theta state for a while before we are in Delta (for example if we wind-down slowly, and are sufficiently relaxed before we fall asleep) then our brains go into a deeper Delta state. In other words, we sleep more soundly. We awake feeling refreshed and rested, and obviously parents enjoy the benefits of this also.

Enjoy this precious time with your child. If it is 5minutes a day, or even just one story a week, these will be times that your little darling will remember and treasure forever, and the benefits they reap will be tremendous.

Benefits of children's meditation

Any form of focus in which to induce relaxation is known as meditation. The benefits of meditation with little ones are exactly the same as they are for adults. Numerous studies have shown that just 5minutes a day or every other day can drastically improve our mental well-being.

Meditation actually releases endorphins - hormones which are responsible for making us feel great. It increases seratonin - our happy hormone in our brain, and the benefits of these working effectively are vast. They include…

- Banishing insomnia
- Beating depression and anxiety
- Bringing focus and clarity to the mind
- Improving concentration
- Increasing creativity
- Creating motivation
- Regulating mood (controlling mood swings)
- Boosting confidence and self esteem
- Making us unconditionally HAPPY!

The physical effects of meditation are astonishing also, it can….

- Lower blood pressure
- Control pain
- Reduce heart rate
- Exercise our lungs in a controlled way (extremely helpful for asthmatics)
- Lower cholesterol
- Reduce muscular tension
- More recent studies have shown that some believe it can even physically change our cellular structure; the power of our mind is incredible.

>>

Benefits to Others

The benefits to parents/carers are obvious. Bedtime will become positive instead of a time of day to be dreaded and the parent/carer/child relationship will vastly improve due to this. Parents will notice that when a child takes time to re-fuel and they are suitably rested they will focus much more deeply, respond more productively and feel happier in general, resulting in contented children and a cheerful atmosphere at home.

The stories are relaxing for the reader also. The fact that they are read slowly naturally slows the reader's breathing. When our breath is relaxed, our bodies relax. Read the stories and relax yourself. Everybody wins.

Relaxation and ADHD/ADD/Aspergers

If you have a child diagnosed with Attention deficit hyperactivity disorder, Attention deficit disorder, or Aspergers syndrome, you may be thinking 'How on Earth could my child possibly sit still long enough to do this?'

However, the results really do speak for themselves…

I spent my earlier years working with children diagnosed with Attention deficit hyperactivity disorder. All extremely highly spirited and challenging little souls. These children taught me so much about the power and incredible strength that we hold in our minds. Simple breathing techniques would instantly calm these children, and they loved doing them, even learning them incredibly quickly.

When I first started writing this book I had these young ones in my mind. You could even say it was they who showed me the real meaning of meditation before I even knew what the word meant. The focus that they would put into their breathing as I talked them through it, just for a few moments, was enough to calm their busy minds and take away the hyperactive feelings and stress that would be whirling around like a crazy cyclone in there. It astonished me.

The stories that follow are short enough to hold the little one's attention, and for the ones who really find it difficult to sit and visualise I have included kiddie calmers such as the breathing meditations (the Red balloon calmer is especially good for when attention is lacking, and the connection is lost between adult and child)

All of the kiddie calmers here increase the child's ability to focus. They practice concentrating without actually being aware that they are doing it. They focus on the visualisation or the breathing technique and naturally train their minds to 'home in' on that subject, therefore extending their concentration span.

Kiddie Calmers

These are techniques to use either on their own to physically and mentally calm your child, or prior to a dreamtime story to prepare your little one for relaxation.

All of the exercises can be taught to your child and used independently by them; for example, when they are at school or in bed trying to sleep, as well as together with you of course. Using these calmers regularly can be a great habit for you and your child to create. They are just as effective on adults also. Choose your favourite and use it at will...

Red Balloon

This is a lovely Kiddie Calmer used to slow breathing and help bring a feeling of total calm.

Find a comfortable place to sit or lie down. Close your eyes…

Now place your hands on your tummy
Imagine there is a red balloon inside it.

Take a long slow breath in, and as you breathe in I want you to imagine the big red balloon in your tummy fills with air and gets bigger- just as a balloon does when you blow it up.

Feel your tummy grow as the pretend red balloon gets bigger…and bigger

Now slowly breathe out.

As you breathe out pretend the balloon is shrinking.
Keep your hands on your tummy. Feel your tummy go down and become smaller as the balloon shrinks.

Can you feel your hands move as your tummy moves in and out?

It grows bigger as you breathe in, and smaller as you breathe out. Just like a balloon.
Isn't that clever?

In… out,
In … out,

Do this for a few minutes. Your mind will feel nice and relaxed and you will feel happy, shiny and new…

When you feel it is time to finish, just open your eyes slowly, wiggle your fingers and your toes, do a big stretch and smile.

Wow! You have just completed a kiddie calmer all by yourself.
Well done, what a star you are!

Tip for grown-ups: This breathing technique is also extremely useful to use during times of constipation. Show your child how to use this when they are sitting on the toilet.

Blow Wind Blow

If you feel cross and angry it is a horrible feeling isn't it.
Would you like to know how to blow it away?

Well it's simple. Just close your eyes, and take in a deep breath.
 Breathe it right down to your toes, as deep as you can.
Then…

BLOOOOOOOW!!!!

Blow your anger across the room with almighty force.
Blow hard, as if you are blowing out ten big birthday candles.

Let's do it again. Are you ready? 1, 2, 3…
BLOOOOOOOW!!!

Goodbye yucky feelings, hello happiness!

Do it as many times as you wish…there, that's better.

Body scrunching

This is a great Kiddie Calmer!
It takes all of that yucky tension that is held in your muscles and throws it away.
Our muscles can feel so tight and tense when we are angry or over-tired, so this is a
perfect exercise to de-stress those muscles and give your body a really nice rest.

First, become comfortable either by lying down or sitting in a cosy chair. Close your
eyes.

Now we will begin by scrunching up all of the muscles in your face...screw your face up
really tightly!
Scrunch up your eyes, and press your lips together.
Now bite your teeth together....
And hold this position for a moment...
Hold it longer still!
Keep holding it!
You can do it...

And relax ...phew! Doesn't that feel good?

Now screw up your hands into a fist, like a ball shape.
Lift your shoulders up toward your ears at the same time.
Do your arms feel really stiff now?
Squeeze your fists hard...
And harder still...
Keep clenching...!
Really squeeze...

And relax... Open your fingers out, relax your hands and let your shoulders rest down.
Feel your arm muscles go soft and floppy. Do your fingers feel relaxed now?

>>

Next, breathe in and pull in your tummy.
Really suck it in…
Hold it!
Keep holding it…
Well done.

Now breathe out.
Let your tummy muscles relax as you breathe out. Doesn't that feel better?

Next, it's time to clench your leg muscles. Point your toes away from you. Feel the tension in your legs…
Hold it!
Hold it longer still…
Keep holding that position…and relax. Let your legs soften and go heavy now. Lovely!

Imagine your whole body just sinks into the bed (or floor or chair). Notice how your body feels now. Does it feel better when your muscles are tense or when they are soft and relaxed?
Doesn't it feel much nicer when your body is relaxed and your muscles are having a rest?

This kiddie calmer shows you the difference between how it feels when your body is tense and how it feels when it is relaxed.
Now you know this technique you can relax your hard working muscles at anytime.

Well done for giving your muscles a break! Phew! They deserve it don't they.

Reeeee - Laaaaax

Find a nice comfortable position, either laying down on the floor, or bed or
sitting up in a comfortable chair…

As you breathe in say ' RE' silently in your head (like this – Reeeee)
Then as you breathe out say 'LAX' quietly in your mind.
So as you are breathing in and out you are telling yourself to 'relax'.
It's as simple as that!

Breathe in – 'Reeeeeee'
Breathe out – 'Laaaaax'
Breathe in – 'Reeeeee'
Breathe out – 'Laaaaax'

And again…

Breathe in – 'Reeeeee'
Breathe out 'Laaaaaaax'
Are you saying the word quietly in your head in time with your breathing?
Re, as you breathe in
Lax as you breathe out

Do it for as long as you like, until you feel nice and calm, and probably quite sleepy too.
Well done!

*Tip for grown-ups: This is a great one for older children's pre-exam nerves as well as a
sleeping aid, or just to quell nerves in any situation. It really works! (On mums and dads
too).*

Dreamtime Stories

These stories are designed to be read aloud by you, the adult, and listened to by your child whilst they close their eyes and use their imagination to visualise themselves taking part in the fun and relaxing story.

Firstly, you should invite your child/ren to become comfortable and relax (maybe use one of the kiddie calmers beforehand if you feel you need to). They then listen to the story and are guided by you to create the scene in their mind. This visualisation technique has been used as a meditation for many years and is extremely successful in creating complete calm and a feeling of utter contentment.

Your child will relish this time spent with you, and adore their new bedtime story. Once they get to know the stories they can take themselves off to these magical places whenever they wish on their own just by using their wonderful imaginations.
During the story allow suitable pauses so that your child has time to imagine each part. I have included pauses to use if you wish. Go with your own instinct and watch your child's reaction so that you can judge how long you wish the pauses to be. A few seconds is normally long enough.

Remember, your child may open their eyes to ask you questions about the story, or to see what is happening as this is new to them. That is fine, just go with them and allow them to do this. Eventually they will become used to listening to their dreamtime story with their eyes closed...

Tip for grown-ups: It is a nice accompaniment to have relaxing music playing softly in the background if you wish. (These can be purchased from many shops on the Internet, simply type 'relaxation music' into your search engine, or look in your local music store)

Kingdom on a cloud

Settle down in comfort, relax your body and close your eyes.

I want you to imagine you are standing in a beautiful garden. Look around you, the grass is green, and there are many colourful flowers here.
(Gentle pause)

Look toward the end of the garden....
You can see a big tall wooden ladder. It reaches up so high you cannot see where it ends. It stretches up, up, up toward the clouds.

You feel very excited, knowing that you are about to have a big adventure.
You start to walk toward the ladder with the feeling of excitement building in your tummy.

See yourself take hold of the wooden ladder. It feels smooth beneath your fingers. Now start to climb the ladder. You feel very safe; you know you will not fall.

Make your way up the ladder now, step by step.
As you become higher you look below you and see the bright colourful flowers in the garden beneath. They look smaller now because you are high above them.

See yourself climbing really high now. Higher...and higher...and higher.
Notice how quiet and calm it is up here in the clouds, feel the warm sunshine on your face as you slowly make your way up the ladder.
(Gentle pause)

Finally, you reach the top. Step carefully from the ladder onto the soft fluffy cloud.
It feels spongy and bouncy.
Feel it with your hands and notice how soft it is, just like cotton wool.

Look in front of you and see a huge red castle amongst the clouds.
How exciting! Coming out of the castle are many little people. They have small wings and are slowly flying toward you.
These are called cherubs.
Watch the little cherubs as they come toward you smiling. Notice how happy they are.

>>

They welcome you to their kingdom and you feel very happy to be here, so safe, relaxed and calm.

One of the cherubs tells you that they live here in the cloud kingdom and they spend their days flying around in the blue sky, looking down at us human beings and making sure that we are safe.

He explains that they also enjoy lying on the clouds listening to the birds singing and feeling the warm sun on their face.

They ask you to relax with them.
You all find a nice comfortable space on the fluffy cloud and lay down.
You sink comfortably into it. Your body feels so calm and cosy in the cloud. It feels like a warm, snuggly blanket, the softest you have ever felt.
(Gentle pause)

Just imagine that you can hear the birds singing, and see the blue sky above you. Think about how this would make you feel.
(Gentle pause)

When you feel it is time to finish relaxing on your cloud, imagine that you are saying goodbye to your cherub friends. See yourself giving them a big hug.
They ask that you promise to do something for them… they ask that every time you look in a mirror, before you do anything else, you must first always say to yourself 'I am GREAT!'
You giggle at this funny request, then nod your head and promise that you will always try to remember this.

Now picture yourself standing up on the cloud and walking towards the top of the ladder that you can just see poking through.

Climb slowly back down the ladder….down, down…. all the way to the ground.

When you reach the bottom, step from the ladder and stand on the grass in your garden. You feel so happy and calm.

Remember, you can visit your cloud kingdom again at anytime. Just use your wonderful mind to take you there.

I hope you enjoyed your time at the Kingdom in the cloud.

Rainbow sliding

Find a comfortable place, relax your body and close your eyes.

Now, as you lie here relaxing I want you to imagine that you are running through a large field. It is a lovely sunny day and as you look around the field you see the green grass, 3 tall trees and a big beautiful blue sky.

You look ahead. Far in front of you, you can see a rainbow.
You stare at the wonderful colours of the rainbow, and can see a bright red rainbow shaped curve, on top of that is sunny yellow, above the yellow is a long curve of pink, then green, then purple, then orange, then blue.
(Gentle pause)

As you look at the great colours you notice that you can actually step onto the rainbow.

You run towards it, excited to touch the beautiful rainbow.
When you reach it, you notice it is huge! It towers high above you.

At the start of the rainbow is a set of steps. Imagine that you can climb the steps to take you to top of the rainbows arch.

You slowly climb all the way to the top of the rainbow.
You feel like a King or Queen high above the field, above everything else.
Take a look at the view around you and notice just how high up you are.
(Gentle pause)

You notice that you can slide all the way down to the other end of the rainbow. Wow! How exciting. Here's a gigantic rainbow slide.

Picture yourself sitting down and imagine you are getting ready to slide.
You know that this is going to be the slide of your life, the biggest, and best, slide ever...

In your mind count to 3...
1, 2, 3
GO!!!

>>

In your mind count to 3…
1, 2, 3
GO!!!

Weeeeeeeeeeeeeeeeeeeeeeeeeeeeeeee !!! sliiiiiiiiiiiiiiiiiiiiiiiide! All the way down…
The wind is whizzing past your ears making a great whooshing sound.
Whooooooosh! Whooooooosh!

You feel free, as if you are flying. It feels great!
Pure happiness and excitement.

weeeeeeeeeeeeeeeeeeeeeeee, you carry on sliding down,
Imagine you are rushing past the trees and feeling the wind on your face as you come to
the end of the rainbow ….

Then you reach the bottom. BUMP!
You lie on the grass feeling so happy.
 Lie there thinking about what you just did. Think about how it felt, and how you feel
right now.

*Tip for grown-ups: Your little one/s can either continue to lie on the grass and relax in
the field, noticing their breathing slowing down as they become more and more calm,
and leave them to slowly drift off to sleep like this.*
Or continue with the story…

Imagine yourself slowly stand up now and you turn and take one last look at your big
colourful rainbow before you walk away through the field.
Picture yourself leaving the field as your rainbow slide story comes to an end.

Know that you can use your rainbow slide in your magic mind whenever you wish.

The magic chair

Find a nice comfortable position. Close your eyes.
Relax, and breathe slowly and deeply.

Just imagine that you are standing in your bedroom, picture what it looks like.
You look towards the middle of the room and notice a red and gold chair that has never been there before.
You look closely at the chair and notice it has a lovely silver pattern around the edge.
You know this is a very special chair.

Imagine yourself sitting down on the chair, and as you do, you notice it gently moves beneath you.
Wooaahh! This must be a magic chair, a real life enchanted chair. How exciting!
I wonder where it will take you?

Suddenly the chair starts to lift you up. It flies slowly towards the window.

The window magically opens wide, and you and the chair fly through it and out into the night air.
Think about how it would feel to sit on this moving chair.
(Gentle pause)

Imagine the air feels cool on your skin as you fly through the sky. You feel completely safe in your chair and know that you will not fall.
Think about how it feels to be up so high in the silent night sky. Notice how calm you feel.
Now imagine you are looking down at the roofs of the houses and the top of the trees, and you see the tiny roads below you.
Use your imagination to think about all the things that you can see.
(Gentle pause)

Watch the twinkling stars above and around you. You see them sparkling, and notice shooting stars whizzing like spirals through the dark sky.
Whizz, Whizz!
It is so lovely up here, there is no noise, no need to move, no need to hurry.
You feel happy and warm inside.
(Gentle pause)

When you feel ready to come home just imagine that you are flying slowly towards your house again. You reach your roof and your magic chair moves downward towards your open bedroom window.
You slowly sit up as the chair takes you in through it and comes to rest on your bedroom floor.

See yourself jump up off your magic chair and then watch it fly back through your bedroom window. It flies off home to its special land, until you wish to call it back and use it again.
Bye bye chair!

Now imagine that you are climbing into your nice comfortable bed. You feel so cosy and warm as you settle down under the covers.
Now keep your eyes closed and get ready to dream of all the wonderful adventures you know you will have when your magic chair comes back to visit you next time.
Goodnight!

Happy Flutter Butterfly

Find a nice comfortable space and lay on your back with your arms by your sides, close your eyes and relax…

Use your imagination to see yourself as a butterfly sitting on a leaf in a wonderful sunny garden.
Just spend a moment thinking about what colour you are. Maybe you are more than one colour, or even multi-coloured.

Just use whichever colours come into your mind, and picture yourself as this beautiful butterfly
(Gentle pause)

Now, imagine yourself fluttering across the garden. You decide that in a moment you will land on the prettiest yellow flower there. (As you flutter you can slowly move your arms up and down if you wish, as if you are really fluttering across the garden)

The flower seems very large because you are so small. Notice how bright it is. The bright sunny colour makes you feel so happy.

Flutter down onto the flower and sit on the pretty petals.

This is the 'Happiness flower'; whenever you kiss the petals you will feel happy all day long. Picture yourself reaching down and kissing the yellow flower.

You feel the warm sun on your wings and hear your bird friends chirping in the distance as you rest on your flower.
(Gentle pause).

Now you decide to spread your wings and flutter across the garden. (Move your arms again slowly if you wish)

>>

See the green grass below you. Feel the wind on your face as you fly around the garden (Gentle pause).

Imagine yourself fluttering down now to land on a beautiful pink flower. Notice how soft the petals feel underneath your tiny butterfly feet.
A buzzy bumblebee stops to land on the same flower next to you. Buzz Buzz.
'Hello Mr Bumblebee' you say.
'Good day Butterfly' he replies.
You both smell the pretty flower petals. It smells so sweet and fresh. 'Mmmm'
This pink flower is 'The flower of calm' and whoever smells it will feel calm and relaxed all day long. Take a big long sniff! Go on!

You decide to set off again and flutter around the garden. (Move your butterfly arms as you lie on the bed if you wish).
As you fly around you spy as a small snail gliding slowly along the garden path. He looks friendly. You are a very happy, calm butterfly as you fly in the sunshiny garden.

It is now time to come down and land again as your adventure ends.
This time you find yourself on the woody branch of a small tree.
 Look around the garden and feel happy as you think about your journey today.
You know that you can come back here at anytime. All you need to do is close your eyes and imagine.

And remember, whenever you wish to feel happy all you have to do is kiss a yellow flower, and smell any pink flower to help you feel calm.

Wow! How does it feel to be a human being again?
I do hope you enjoyed being a butterfly.

Crazy-coloured Jungle Snake

Close your eyes, relax, and make your body
comfortable, take 3 long, slow deep breaths, and relax …

Use your clever imagination and see yourself in a large, exciting looking jungle.
It has big tall trees with brightly coloured strange looking fruits hanging from them, and big
tropical birds singing and shouting loudly "Squawk Squawk!"

The jungle is a very hot sticky place and you feel hotter and hotter as you walk through
it…

Suddenly you hear a loud booming voice behind you "HELLO! WOULD YOU LIKE
TO COOL DOWN?"
You spin around and there you see a HUGE CRAZY-COLOURED JUNGLE SNAKE.
It is GIGANTIC!!!
It has big bold colours all over its giant body. Stripes of brilliant red and blue, with
green, yellow and orange spots. His googly eyes are large and his smile is wide.
You know that he is a friendly snake and you nod your head and agree, "Yes please, I
would really like to cool down Mr crazy coloured jungle snake"
"THEN HOP ON" He booms and waves his tail in the air.

You climb aboard the snake's back and feel so high.

He begins to slither, slowly at first, then faster and faster across the jungle floor and you
feel the wind rush into your face as you move so quickly.
Your hands grip the snakes back.
 Hold on tight!

Picture yourself whizzing through the jungle now, past the trees, past the bright loud
squawking birds and past the swinging monkeys who chatter chatter chatter!

>>

Your hair blows in the wind as the snake zooms along and you feel cool and refreshed. Faster and faster and faster he goes.

The wind rushes louder and louder in your ears. You are having so much fun!
Just imagine how exciting this is, and see yourself laughing with your new snake friend
(Gentle pause)

"It is time to sssslow down now," Hisses the crazy-coloured jungle snake.
Gradually he begins to slow down and glides smoothly through the jungle.

You decide to lay down on his back and enjoy the journey.
You are relaxing now as the snake sneaks slowly and silently across the ground.
The birds are quieter, and the monkeys have stopped chattering.

You feel calm and so relaxed as you enjoy your comfortable ride. Think of all the sights that you see as you watch the jungle pass by.
Feel happy and peaceful as you imagine yourself there.
Notice how calm your body feels as you enjoy your ride.
(Gentle pause)

Now it is time for you to say goodbye to your colourful snake friend.
He stops, and you carefully slide from his back. "Thank you crazy-coloured jungle snake" You say.
"Anytime my friend, anytime". He answers.
Watch him glide away as he gently and slowly moves through the jungle on his soft crazy coloured belly.

You know that you can see your colourful friend again whenever you wish. Just use your imagination and take your clever mind off to the jungle and your crazy-coloured jungle snake will always be waiting.

Fairy Forest Adventure

Find a nice comfortable place, Close your eyes and relax your body...

There are many fairies in the forests. If you imagine hard enough you can take your mind there and meet them.

Use your imagination to see yourself in a lovely forest full of tall green leafy trees. You are standing in front of a big old tree right in the middle of the forest.

If you look above you, you can see the big blue sky and the yellow shining sun, and white fluffy clouds float past the tops of the trees.
(Gentle pause)

As you start to walk through the forest, past the trees and flowers you hear the birds singing above you, they are sitting in the branches way up high. Their happy song makes you smile.
You look ahead and see a little white rabbit hop among the flowers. Hop, hop, hop!
With your eyes closed just imagine these wonderful sights for a moment.
(Gentle pause)

Suddenly you hear a rustling in the bushes and out jumps a small fairy. She is tiny with a pretty yellow dress, delicate pink wings and wispy red hair. She looks up at you and smiles. You cannot believe your eyes. A fairy! Right here in front of you.

She walks towards you. Put out your hand and watch her hop onto it.
She asks you to meet her pixie friends and of course, you agree.

Your fairy friend leads you to a big oak tree and shows you a red door just large enough for you to squeeze through.

>>

Picture yourself going through the door and you see that inside is a round room filled with little tables and chairs. The sight astounds you as you see the pixies and fairies sitting at the tables eating a feast of jam treacle sandwiches and honeyberry pies.
 Now, spend a moment picturing the scene. What does the room look like? Imagine what the fairy folk are wearing?

You notice that your fairy friends are calling you, inviting you to sit down with them. Think about how they sound and how they look. See the feast on the table and imagine what it tastes like.
(Gentle pause)

You can hear music playing in the room amongst the chatter of the woodland folk. Notice how you feel as you sit in this happy place with your new smiling friends listening to music and having fun.
Maybe think about what you would like to say to the fairies and pixies and listen to their replies.
Use your imagination, let it run free.
(Gentle pause)

You feel so happy here. The fairy folk are your friends, enjoy your time in the tree room, laughing, smiling and eating with them.
(Gentle pause)

Now it is time to leave the special tree and your fairy friends.
You shake their hands and give them gentle hugs, then say goodbye and walk away.
Squeeze back through the red door and out into the sunny forest.
See yourself walk past the trees and the pretty flowers dancing in the breeze.
 "Goodbye White rabbit" you say as he appears again and hops gently passed your feet.

You feel happy as you leave the forest, knowing that you can visit your magical fairy friends again whenever you wish.
They are always here; sometimes we just cannot see them with our eyes open.

Dolphin dreams

Find a nice comfortable place and relax your body, take 3 nice, long, deep breaths...

Picture yourself walking along a lovely sunny beach. The sand is soft and warm under your feet and you can feel the sun kissing your face as you look up to the sky.

You walk towards the sea and dip your feet into the water.
It feels fresh and cool.

Now imagine that you are looking out into the ocean and notice two playful noses bobbing up and down in the water.
You realise they belong to two dolphins who are swimming gently towards you.
Watch them glide through the water.
They swim to you with their little tails swishing in the sea inviting you in.
They want you to play with them. You feel calm and know that no harm will come to you.

See yourself run, splish-splashing into the water towards them. The water feels lovely, you smile and laugh, this is so much fun!
Now you are swimming towards the amazing dolphins.

Notice their beautiful eyes gazing at you, and their large smiles as they chat gleefully.

Suddenly they swim along side you. Imagine yourself reaching out and touching their warm skin.

Put your arms out and gently hug them. Give them both a big snuggly cuddle.
Feel the love flowing from the dolphins to you.
You can feel their magic.
(Gentle pause)

>>

Now imagine that you are diving deep, deep down under the sea and swimming along with the dolphins, twisting and turning, gathering speed as you swim easily with these wonderful friends.

Think about how this feels for a moment - swimming faster and faster under the water, breathing easily as if by magic, feeling the safest you have ever felt.
See yourself now…faster…and faster…AND FASTER. Wow! This is so exciting!!!
(Gentle pause)

Now it is time to slow down and just glide through the water with the dolphins.Just relax, Swim slowly and gently with them now, playing and laughing with your new friends.

Feel their soft, silky heads and their smooth fins.
Watch their tails dance as they dip and swerve around you.
Look into their eyes and see the love that they have for you.
Feel happy that you are spending time with them.

Now it is time to leave your dolphin friends. Until next time.

You slowly swim back to the seashore and stand on the sand.
Feel the lovely sun on your face once more.
You turn around and wave at your two friends. 'Goodbye!' you call.
They wave their shiny, long noses at you and open their mouths in a big smile.
Bye bye dolphins.
You can use your clever mind to visit your dolphins again whenever you wish.
Maybe one day you can draw a picture of your dolphin friends!

Splishy splashy rain

Tip for Grown-ups: This is a dreamtime story with a difference. Hou could even say it is a 'wideawake story' instead.
It is to be used whenever your child needs some extra cheer or energy. It is revitalising and exciting rather than relaxing and never fails to win a big smile. When carried out with siblings or in a group setting this is a great confidence booster and bonds the group perfectly.
It is good fun to act it out as you read it aloud and stand up with your child jumping in and out of the puddles. Enjoy!

Either close your eyes, become comfortable and imagine that you are standing in a nice big splashy puddle OR you can stand up with your eyes open and use your imagination to have fun splishy, splashy, sploshing around…

Look down and see bright shiny red wellington boots on your feet.
Splash one foot in a big puddle, hear the sound and watch the water.
Splish Splosh, Splish Splosh!
Now splash the other foot…Splash, Splish, Splosh!

Feel raindrops falling on your head and down your face. They splash onto your nose.
The rain feels warm, not cold. It feels just like a lovely shower.
Lift your face up to the sky and feel the rain bouncing onto it.
(Gentle pause)

WOW! As the raindrops land on your skin you notice that they are golden.
Watch the sparkly raindrops land on your arms.
This magical rain brings you excitement with each drop. It fills you with joy and makes you smile.
Splishy Splashy golden raindrops!
As they splash onto your head, they bounce onto the floor - filling the golden puddle and making it bigger.

Stamp your feet in the puddle. See the golden water spray as you splash faster and faster, stamping harder and harder.
Laugh as you kick the puddle and splash the water all around you.
Kick, Kick, Kick.

>>

You laugh as more and more happy, sparkly raindrops fall from the sky and soak you wet through - filling you with joy.
See yourself laughing loudly! You laugh and laugh until you think you'll never stop.
Splash Splash Splash.
Splish, Splosh, Splash.

Then you look up in the sky above and see the rain shower gently stop.
Goodbye sparkly, golden rain shower .
Drip, Drop, Drip, Drop

Have one last cheeky splash in the puddle…a big huge jump. Then walk away from it.
Was that fun? I bet it was. How do you feel now? Happy? Excited? And probably quite wet I bet.

Final thought

Relaxation time is the most beautiful, pampering gift that you can give to yourself. Allowing yourself valuable 'You time' will benefit your mental, emotional, physical and spiritual health, as well as those around you; the positive effects really are contagious. If children learn this now, they will grow up automatically scheduling 'Me time' into their diaries. Therefore, by taking control of their own well-being they will know how to deal with stress as it comes. By prioritising time for relaxation they will grow into calm, confident and capable adults

As my eldest Son has grown, I have advanced from reading him dreamtime stories to meditating with him. It really is not about spending hours chanting in uncomfortable positions, we just simply spend some quiet time together once in a while listening to the birds outside or visualising a colour floating in front of our closed eyes for fun, just to see what our imaginations can do and remind us of how clever our minds are.

He is a calm, grounded child with a focused mind and a knack for problem solving. By using relaxation techniques he naturally solves his own sleep problems and other stresses. This has given him confidence in himself and his abilities.
Please understand that sometimes my Son is a normal, teenage grump- monster who loves his game consoles as much as any other twelve year old, but now and again he will prise himself away and 'just be' and it is this combination that makes him the special person he is.

Even my three year old enjoys relaxing time. He enjoys using deep breathing techniques which he practices to help his sometimes upset stomach, and The red balloon is his favourite calmer which he uses himself before sleep. It is beautiful to watch him do this naturally now whenever he feels the need, and the deeper sleep is invaluable to him and myself and my husband also.

They have the power within them to relax, soothe or revive themselves, even to heal pain, just by focusing their minds on their breath, or visualising a calming colour or picture in their mind
I hope this book will start your little angel on the road to relaxation and meditation so that they can unlock their own potential and discover this fantastic way of being.
Once our tiny ones realise the power of their precious little minds they really will become the supremely confident beings that we wish them to be and therefore have the power to follow the lives that we wish them to lead.

Acknowledgments to the little legends

The most important people to thank for helping me in the making of this book are of course, the children.
They are our teachers. From the first moment that I started working with children when I was fifteen years old I knew they would be my inspiration throughout my life.
Their pure innocence and trust is something we should aim to get back to. Society has become so cynical and distrustful of our fellow human beings. Notice the way a child instantly starts to play with its peer in a playground with no awkward introductions needed. They just trust that this small fellow stranger will accept them.

Look at the way they embrace everything with such excitement…a rain shower is seen as a fun distraction on their journey home instead of a hindrance, and a bumblebee in the garden will become an intriguing friend, rather than a nuisance.
Everything is full of wonder because the world viewed through a child's eyes is a world seen as the adventure that it is.

I watch my little ones delight at new experiences and I learn to do the same. If a flower catches their eye they will stop to admire it, not hurry pass.
Life is full of excitement. The positives will always outshine the negatives if we look for them just as little ones do. Maybe we could stop and smell the roses too.

Children are full of love, unconditional love. There are no egos involved, no conditions. They know how to 'Just be'. They are themselves; they do not pretend to be someone they are not just to make another warm to them.
They are free.

So I must thank the very first child that ever showed me this way of being, and all the others in between, right up to this current day.
I am blessed to sit and watch my own children play as they teach me unknowingly about life, and how to live it.

And finally, I most definitely cannot forget to say a big thank you to my wonderful Son Ollie who wrote the Forest Fairy and Splishy Splashy stories.
And to all the Children - our teachers on this planet. Continue to shine your light and illuminate our path. Thank you.

Lightning Source UK Ltd.
Milton Keynes UK
UKOW021949050313

207199UK00011B/589/P